STUART MCALEESE

Fit for The West Highland Way

Getting Fit For Your First 100 Mile Backpacking Trip

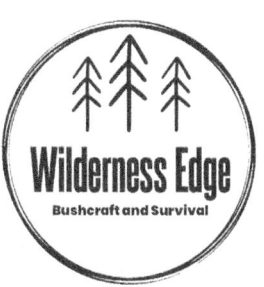

First published by Wilderness Edge 2024

Copyright © 2024 by Stuart McAleese

All rights reserved. No part of this publication may be reproduced, stored or transmitted in any form or by any means, electronic, mechanical, photocopying, recording, scanning, or otherwise without written permission from the publisher. It is illegal to copy this book, post it to a website, or distribute it by any other means without permission.

Stuart McAleese asserts the moral right to be identified as the author of this work.

First edition

This book was professionally typeset on Reedsy.
Find out more at reedsy.com

Contents

1	Introduction	1
2	Programme Overview	6
3	Programme Specifics	8
4	Mental Training	15
5	Developing Mental Toughness through Training	21
6	Nutritional Guidance	22
7	Recovery and Recuperation	25
8	Injuries	32
9	General Advice on When to Seek Professional Help	38
10	Training Programme	39
11	Conclusion	52

1

Introduction

Welcome to The West Highland Way fitness guide. My name is Stuart McAleese and I'm extremely excited to be writing this book!

I have had a long relationship with the West Highland Way over the years. Like many aspiring long distance backpackers, it was the first 100 mile backpacking trip I did. I walked it solo in about 8 days. As I walked into Fort William I was blistered, sunburned, covered in midge bites and absolutely knackered.

But I had fallen in love! The love affair for long distance hiking was born on that trip and it's one of my proudest achievements. Since then I have walked thousands of miles on various trails - both recognised and self charted - across the world in countries like the United States, Greenland, Andorra, Iceland, Norway, Peru, Ireland, Wales and England.

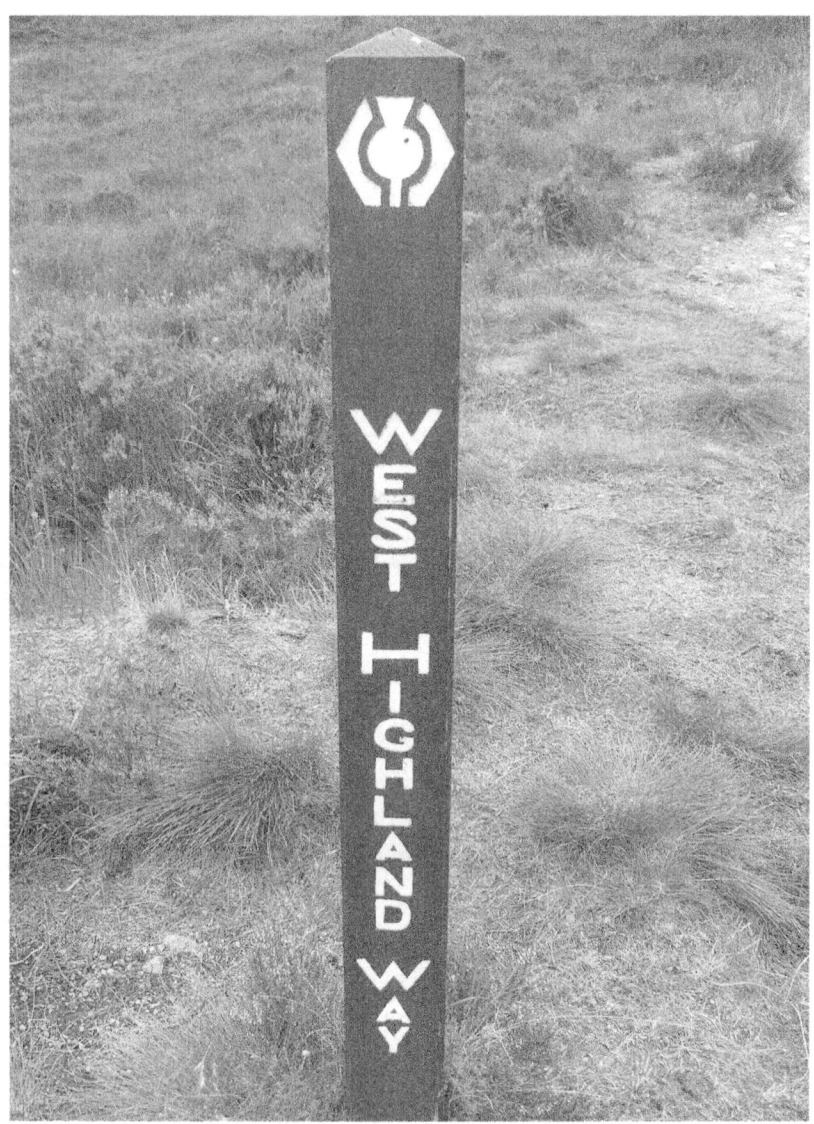

But I also returned to the West Highland Way many other times. I've hiked it in every season. I used it as a highway to get to and from the many mountains close to the trail which I have climbed. In 1993 a good

INTRODUCTION

friend and I attempted to backpack it as fast as we could. He had to pull out with a knee injury but I did the full West Highland Way in two days. Tired is an understatement! In 2003 I attempted to run it in under 24 hours but failed and had to pull out at Tyndrum.

I've also had the pleasure of sharing the experience with others. My late wife and I had a great time walking the West Highland Way on our first holiday as a couple. My sisters both walked it as have many friends.

Then in 1996 I funded my way through university (I returned to education at the ripe old age of 26) by working for various providers and adventure travel companies as a trial guide. Over the next four summers I walked the West Highland Way approximately 24 times guiding over 200 individuals. So I know the route pretty well.

As a guide I got many questions from clients as the departure date came closer. Many are those you would expect - which size of rucksack, which brand of midge repellent, what boots, how many days rain can be expected. But the most common questions were around how to prepare physically for the West Highland Way. I understand that. Pulling on a rucksack loaded with your shelter, bedroom, kitchen, wardrobe and everything else, and then to walk for 100 miles through the wilds of Scotland is not a normal thing to do. Life doesn't really prepare you for it.

Even if life, job and regular workouts do provide a base, it's quite a specific activity. To carry 30lbs to 50lbs for seven to ten days, all day, every day, across uneven ground, up and down hill, in rain, hail and sun (sometimes all in the same hour!!) is not normal.

I found that out of the hundreds of people I've guided, and hiked with on other trials, that the ones who get the most enjoyment and finish injury free (not counting blisters as injury) are the ones who prepared. Benjamin Franklin said that 'by failing to prepare, you are preparing to fail'.

Wise words.

This guide is an attempt to help you prepare for your own West Highland Way hike.

But this isn't just for the West Highland Way.

There are many hikes and backpacking trips of about a week's duration or 100 miles which this guide can help you prepare for. The principles and what you learn here are as applicable to the Cumbrian Way as they are to West Highland Way.

Over the next few sections I'm going to run over what this guide is, and what it's not. We will look at training goals, kit required and how the programme is broken down. Then we'll look at nutrition, mental training, stress management and sleep as well as what to do if you get injured. I'll cover some frequently asked questions people have had then we get to the training programme itself.

With all that said, let's get started!

INTRODUCTION

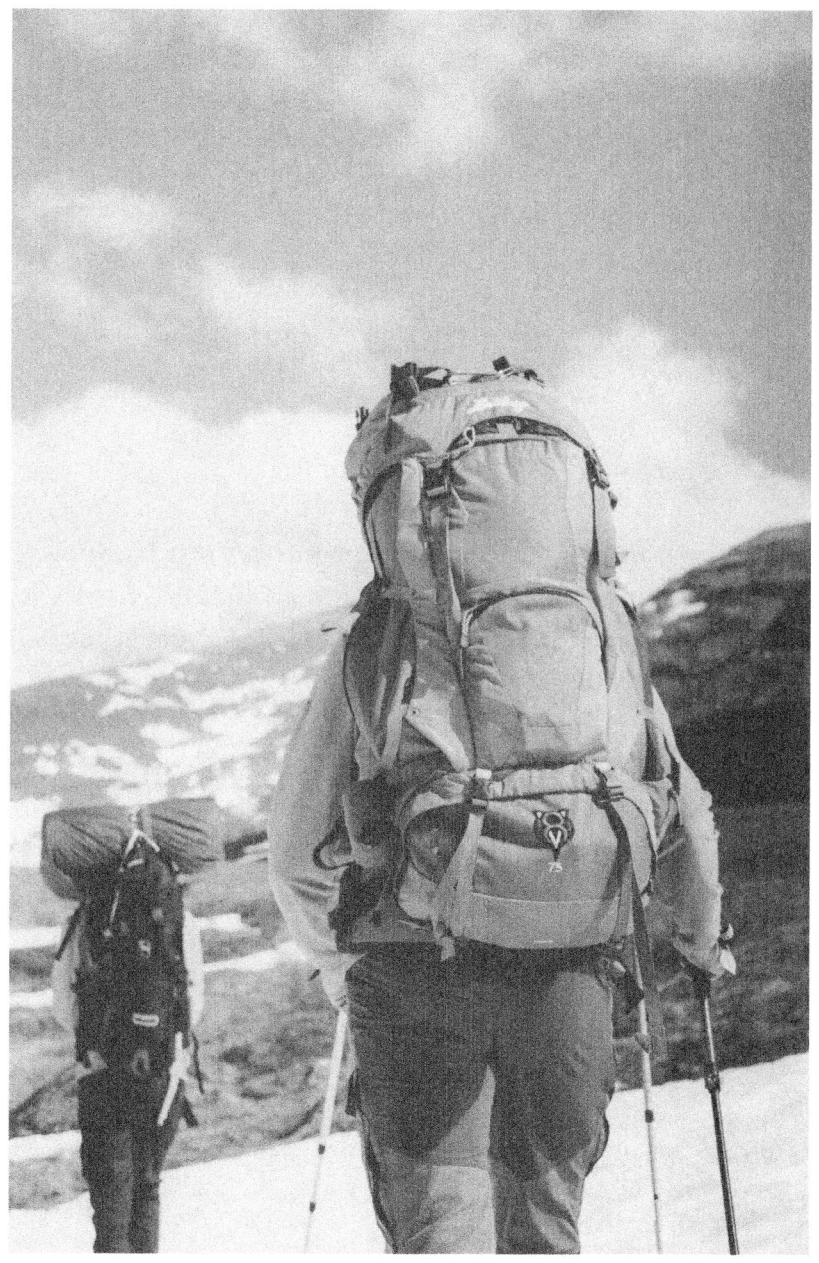

2

Programme Overview

In a nutshell, this programme is designed to prepare a fairly novice backpacker to be able to carry a rucksack of between 30lbs and 50lbs on a trip lasting seven to ten days and assuming they will walk from ten to fifteen miles a day.

Fairly novice? I assume you have done at least one overnight under canvas. I assume you have the kit you need for this. It may not be the most expensive, the best branded or the lightest. But you have the kit you need to walk all day, pitch up, cook a meal, deal with any minor medical events and then get up and walk the next day.

I am also assuming you have the basic skills required - you can navigate, you can sort blisters, you can cook.

This is a demanding programme. It's not at all easy and will require commitment and dedication on your part to complete it and get the most out of it.

As an aside, what if you aren't backpacking? What if you are walking using serviced accommodation, baggage transport and such so you are simply carrying a day pack. Will this programme help? Without a doubt. Being physically prepared has so many advantages nad will always enhance your trip.

Let's briefly look at what this guide is not. This is not designed to provide information on the following:

- A detailed overview of the route itself;
- What kit you need;
- Logistics;
- What to eat;
- Best boots, waterproofs, tents, sleeping bags, sleeping mats;
- Good photography locations;
- Local flora and fauna;
- Local history;
- Travel ot the start of the back from the end;
- Accommodation on the way.

It's about getting as fit as you can within a specific time period in order to increase your chances of success on The West Highland Way.

3

Programme Specifics

Programme Goals
This programme is designed with the overall aim of getting you in shape to complete The West Highland Way and to aid in you enjoying it. That's the high level, key aim of this text. However, there are smaller aims within that, elements which make this a specific programme rather than a general training plan.

These are:

- To develop a high level of hiking and backpacking endurance to allow you to complete the daily and weekly averages required, under load, to complete your hike on The West Highland Way or a similar route;
- To build strength and endurance in your legs and feet to withstand the daily grind along the trail. This will harden the legs and feet to the stresses you will encounter;
- To develop the specific muscular endurance and movement patterns to allow uphill movement with a pack on and to not encounter undue stress, fatigue or injury;

- To strengthen your upper body so the pack won't feel unduly heavy on your trip; and
- To prepare your core for the effort of carrying a loaded pack for a week or longer.

Exercise Equipment Requirements

This is a proverbial can of worms! I am keen that you don't have to spend a lot of money on kit should you train at home. Should you train in a commercial gym you should be able to do what you need there as well. It's a balance.

The kit requirements are modest but there are some things you will need. If you chose to train at home and need kit you don't have, then try purchasing second hand.

You will need:

- A pair of dumbbells or kettlebells - 14kg for men and 10kg for women;
- A sandbag - 20kg for men, 15kg for woman;
- A step, bench or box for step ups. No higher than 18inches;
- A pack for training with. Ideally use the pack you will use on The West Highland Way. load it with 30lbs and have additional weight to take it up to 40lbs;
- A foam roller for recovery work.

All of these are available in commercial gyms.

If training at home, the one item which sl likely to be harder ot get is a sandbag. These can be purchased second hand. I got mine in Aldi for not much at all.

Time Requirements

You have a life. Job. family. Social life. Maybe kids. Perhaps a demanding schedule. They key thing with time is that your prep should not take over your entire life. Each workout is designed to be completed in 60 - 90 minutes.

The longer rucks will take more time. And you will need to hike for 3 - 4 hours one day a week.

Always take one day a week completely off to recover.

Programme Timing

The programme is built across a 6 week period. Do the programme so you have the six week programme, then a week of rest while you pack kit and get ready for The West Highland Way and then do it. Like this:

Week - 8: Get training kit ready, pack your ruck, check out the gym if you are using one
   Week - 7: Week 1 of the programme
   Week - 6: Week 2 of the programme
   Week - 5: Week 3 of the programme
   Week - 4: Week 4 of the programme
   Week - 3: Week 5 of the programme
   Week - 2: Week 6 of the programme
   Week -1: Rest and kit pack
   Week 0: West Highland Way

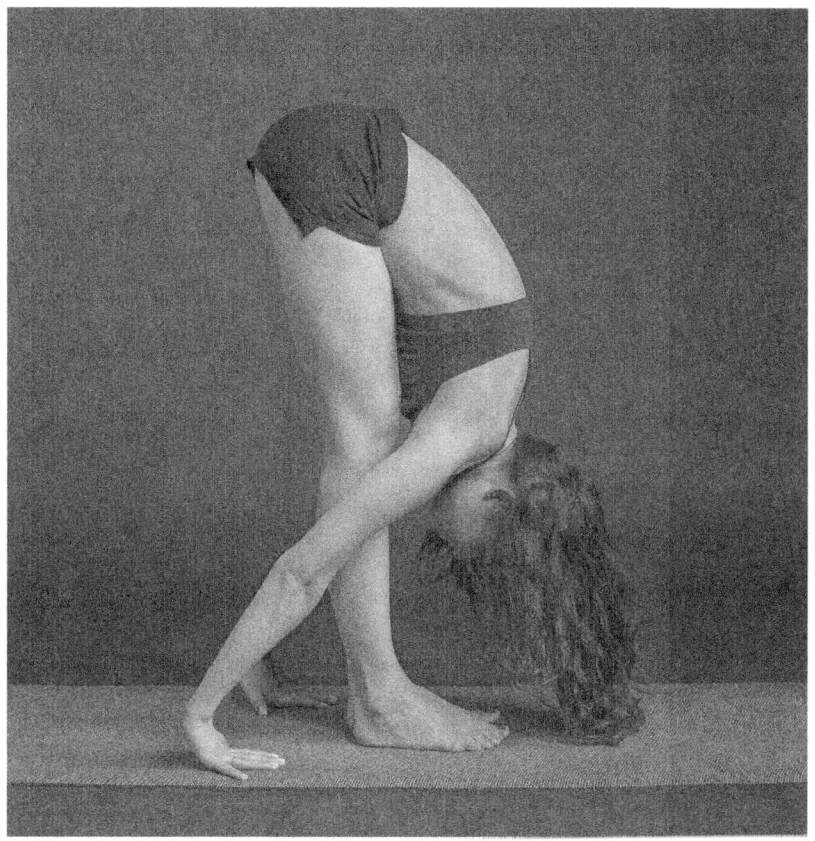

If you want to train for longer, follow the programme through to the completion of Week 5. Then alternate Week 4 and Week 5 for as long as you need. It's hard on the body so I wouldn't recommend any longer than 4 cycles of this.

Programme Cadence
    Over the week, the programme is broken down as follows:

Monday: Step ups and calf raise intervals
    Tuesday: Strength and a light jog or walk

Wednesday: Moderate Ruck
Thursday: Step ups and calf raise intervals
Friday: Strength and a light jog or walk
Saturday: Long Ruck
Sunday: Rest

As you can see, its very simple but, believe me, it's brutally effective.

<u>Activity Selection</u>

The programme has been developed with the following activities as they are the ones which will get you the best results due to how specific they are for trails like The West Highland Way. These are:

Step Ups. These are a basic exercise which best replicate going uphill under load. They are tough and hard and it is a grind. But they will prepare you well for ascending Conic Hill, The Devils Staircase out of Glencoe and the 250m ascent out of Kinlochleven.

Use a step, a bench, a box. Ideally outside and do these in any weather. If it's raining, put your waterproofs on. Put on the boots you plan to wear on The West Highland Way.

You will do thousands of these over the course of the programme. Not only do they build physical strength in your legs and feet, they build mental stamina as well.

One way of keeping count of how many you have done is to take small stones in your hand. Pick up one for each 100 steps. When you complete 100 steps, drop the stone.

Rucking. Back in the day we used the word 'hiking' for this. In the military, we called it 'yomping'. Now it's a sport all on its own and it's called 'rucking'. So, put on your pack, dress appropriately, wear your boots and walk.

The Moderate Ruck on Wednesday can be done around you home, to or from work etc. Just get the miles in.

The Long Ruck on the Saturday is ideall y done in the countryside on similar trails to the West Highland Way. this should resemble, as closely, what you will encounter on the hike.

Calf Raises. Research has found an interval training method called Tabatha works very effectively at conditioning muscles and lungs.

The first muscles to go when you move uphill or over a longer distance are the calf muscles. So, calf raises done in a Tabatha sequence will focus on this area.

You do this exercise unloaded - so your bodyweight only. Stand on a step and for 20 seconds of calf raises. Then hold in the high extension point - so in the upper raise point. Hold for 10 seconds. That's one round. Do eight rounds continuously. It's only four minutes but it will smoke your calves.

Upper Body Strength and Core. Although The West Highland Way is mainly a lower body activity, we need to ensure that you have good upper body strength so you don't get injured and so that you don't get unduly fatigued carrying a loaded back.

Some simple kettlebell or dumbbell circuits will take care of this. Core work is simple - full body planks. Not easy. But simple.

Speed Walk or Jog. A supplemental exercise to keep activity levels high and build overall endurance. If you like to run or jog, then do that. If you don't, then simply walk fast. Do this unloaded. Working on a treadmill is fine.

If you don't know what the exercises are, there's plenty on YouTube to watch.

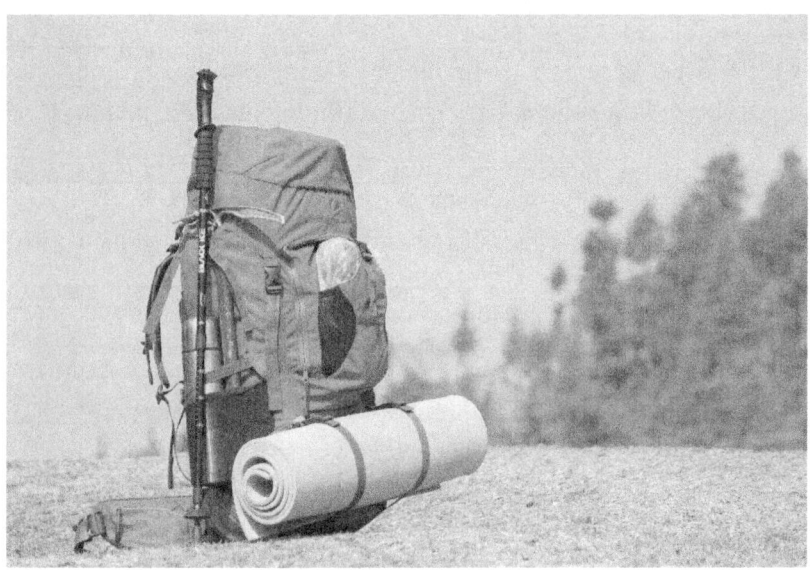

4

Mental Training

Hiking 100 miles is a formidable physical challenge, but it is equally a test of mental toughness. Mental toughness involves several key components such as goal setting, resilience, visualisation, managing demotivation on the trail, and developing mental toughness through pre-trek training. This holistic approach is essential to conquer such a daunting task.

Goal Setting

The journey of a thousand miles begins with a single step, but it is the goals set along the way that provide the direction and motivation. Setting goals is fundamental in preparing for a 100-mile hike. Goals should be SMART: Specific, Measurable, Achievable, Relevant, and Time-bound.

Specific goals define exactly what you want to achieve. For instance, "I want to hike 100 miles on The West Highland Way." This goal is clear and unambiguous. Smaller training goals may be to hike a specific 12 mile walk on Saturday, to reduce the time to do 700 step ups, to feel more comfortable caring the pack you will on The West Highland Way.

Measurable goals allow you to track progress. Breaking down the 100 miles into daily targets based on where you are camping makes the goal measurable.

Achievable goals are realistic and attainable. While aiming for 100 miles is ambitious, ensuring that daily targets are within your physical capacity is crucial.

Relevant goals align with your broader objectives and passions. If you love nature and seek adventure, a 100-mile hike is relevant.

Time-bound goals set a deadline, which in this case is completing The West Highland Way. This urgency helps maintain focus and drive.

Resilience

Resilience is the ability to bounce back from setbacks and continue pushing forward despite difficulties. On a 100-mile hike, hikers face numerous challenges such as harsh weather, physical exhaustion, injuries, and mental fatigue. Developing resilience is essential to overcome these obstacles.

Building resilience starts with embracing a positive attitude. Adopting a growth mindset, where challenges are seen as opportunities for growth rather than insurmountable obstacles, fosters resilience. For instance, encountering a steep incline can be reframed as an opportunity to strengthen leg muscles and test endurance.

Preparation also plays a critical role in building resilience. Training hikes that simulate the conditions of The West Highland Way can prepare the mind and body for the actual challenge. Learning from each training hike and improving strategies for coping with difficulties strengthens resilience.

Some people find having a group of friends around them helps. You can lean on them for encouragement and support as thy can with you.

Visualisation

Visualisation is a powerful mental technique that involves creating a mental image of successfully completing The West Highland Way. This practice can enhance motivation, focus, and performance.

Visualisation should be vivid and detailed. Picture yourself at various stages of the hike: starting out with enthusiasm, overcoming obstacles with determination, and finally reaching the 100-mile mark with a sense of accomplishment. Incorporating all senses in the visualisation – the sounds of nature, the smell of fresh air, the feel of the trail beneath your feet – makes the experience more real and impactful.

Regular visualisation sessions can reinforce the belief in your ability to complete The West Highland Way. It helps in mentally rehearsing responses to potential challenges, such as how to stay calm during heavy rain or push through when fatigue sets in. This mental rehearsal builds confidence and prepares the mind for the journey ahead.

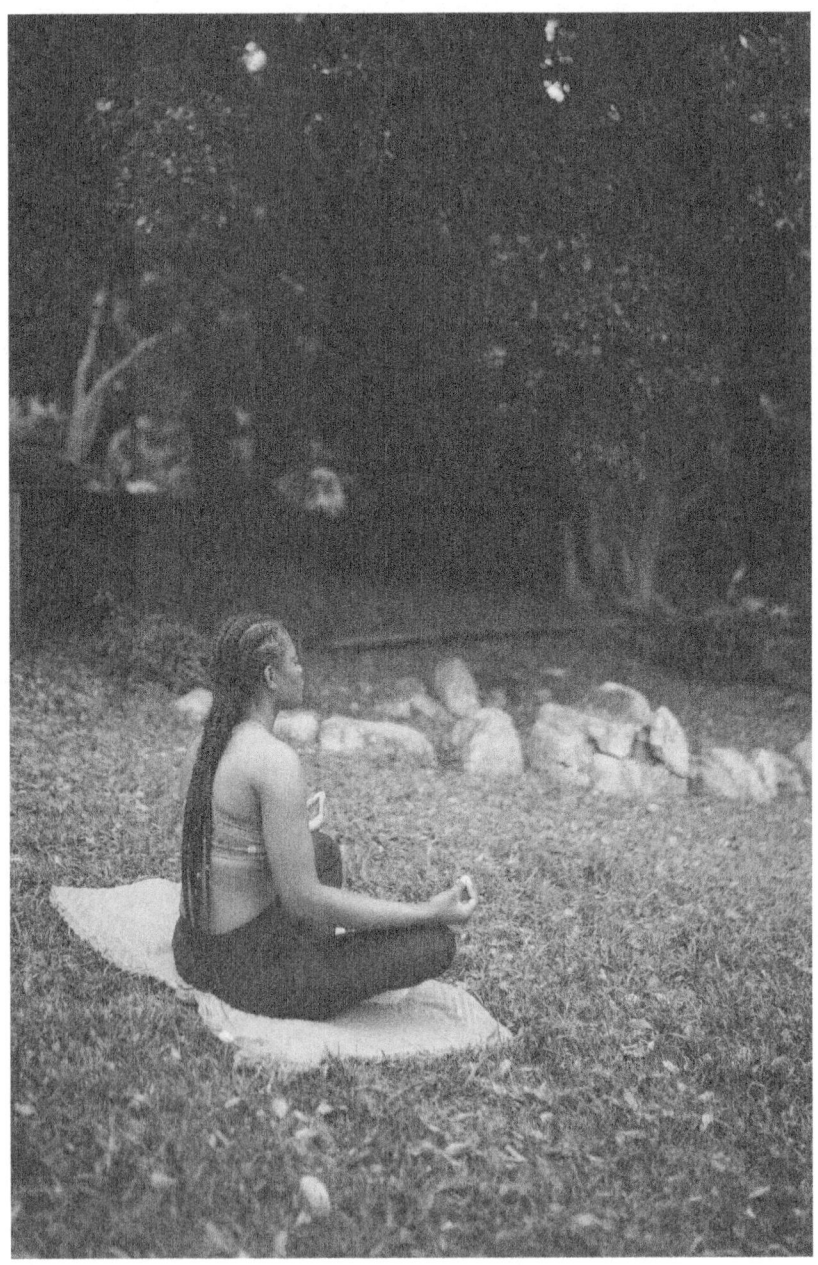

Managing Demotivation on the Trail

Demotivation is inevitable on a long hike, especially during tough sections or when faced with continuous challenges. Managing demotivation is crucial to keep moving forward.

One effective strategy is maintaining a positive inner dialogue. Self-talk can significantly impact motivation. Replacing negative thoughts with positive affirmations, such as "I am strong" or "I can do this," can help sustain motivation. Additionally, connecting with fellow hikers or support networks through social media can provide encouragement and a sense of camaraderie.

Taking care of physical needs is also essential for managing demotivation. Ensuring proper nutrition, hydration, and rest can prevent physical exhaustion from contributing to mental fatigue. Regular breaks to stretch and refuel can rejuvenate both body and mind.

Developing Mental Toughness through Training

Mental toughness can be cultivated through deliberate practice and training before The West Highland Way. Pre-trek training should encompass mental preparation.

Mental Preparation: Mental training can be incorporated into physical workouts. Techniques such as mindfulness meditation and controlled breathing can enhance focus and stress management. Mindfulness practice helps in staying present and reducing anxiety about the challenges ahead.

Simulation of Challenges: Pre-trek training should include simulations of potential challenges. Hiking in adverse weather conditions, tackling difficult terrains, and practising long-duration hikes can prepare the mind for the unpredictability of the trail. Reflecting on these experiences and learning coping strategies builds mental toughness.

Journaling and Reflection: Keeping a journal to document training progress, challenges faced, and lessons learned can be a powerful tool. Reflecting on past experiences and recognizing growth fosters a sense of achievement and resilience. This practice can also highlight areas that need further improvement, allowing for targeted training.

Professional Guidance: Seeking guidance from experienced hikers or professional coaches can provide valuable insights and motivation. They can offer tips on mental strategies, training routines, and practical advice for the trail. Engaging in workshops or group training sessions can also provide a sense of community and support.

5

Developing Mental Toughness through Training

6

Nutritional Guidance

This can be a proverbial can of worms. These nutritional guidelines are from my own experience. I really have to stress this - I am **NOT** a nutritionist, health care professional, medical professional, dietician, doctor or anything. These guidelines are simply some things you may decide to try based on your own circumstances.

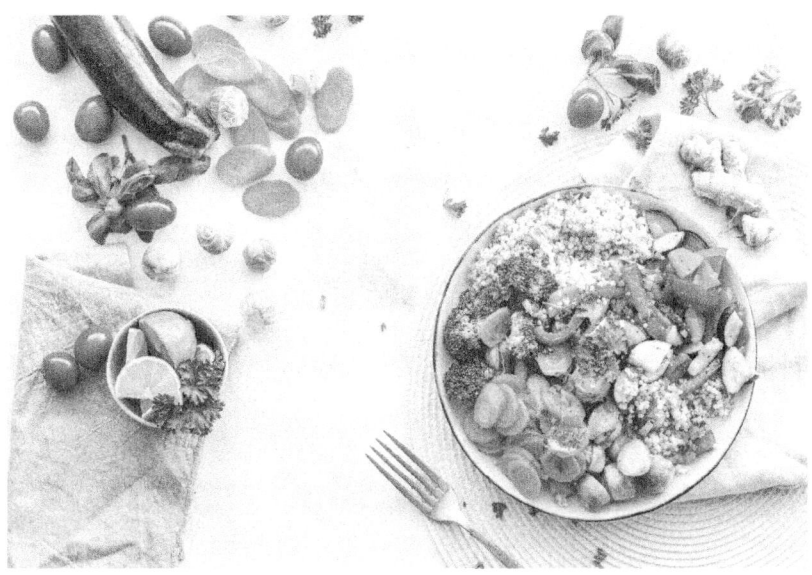

So, my guidance:

- Do as your health care professional suggests especially if you have a medical condition. I personally have Ulcerative Colitis triggered by gluten and dairy. So my first focus in on what I can eat with my condition. Do the same.
- Balance. A wide range of foods exist. Be balanced. Eating only one food group causes problems in other areas.
- Colour. East as much colour as you can. This will, generally, equate to a wide variety of food groups.
- Hydrate. And hydrate. And hydrate. Lots of water.
- Protein with every meal. It will make you feel fuller for longer. How much? Some recommendations are 1g of protein for 1lb of bodyweight. That is excessive for most people so go for half that.
- AVOID UPF.
- Does it matter what diet you follow? Vegan. Vegetarian. Pescatarian.

Carnivore, Keto. Paleo. Not all all.
- Practice feeding strategies for the trail. When you are doing your training rucks, take some snacks which you may use on The West Highland Way and see how they go down.

7

Recovery and Recuperation

Recovery from heavy training volumes is a critical component of any athletic regimen, allowing the body to heal, adapt, and ultimately improve performance. Various recovery methods, including active recovery, stretching, yoga, massage, ice baths, contrast showers, saunas, and proper hydration, can facilitate this process. Understanding Delayed Onset Muscle Soreness (DOMS) is also essential in managing recovery effectively.

Active Recovery

Active recovery involves engaging in low-intensity exercise following intense training sessions. This approach helps maintain blood flow to muscles, promoting nutrient delivery and waste removal, which aids in muscle repair and reduces stiffness.

Examples of Active Recovery:

- **Light jogging or walking**: This can be particularly beneficial after high-impact activities like running or weightlifting.

- **Swimming**: Provides a full-body workout with minimal joint strain, making it ideal for recovery.
- **Cycling at a low intensity**: This helps to keep the legs moving without significant exertion.

Active recovery should be performed at a conversational pace, ensuring it does not add further stress to the body but rather facilitates relaxation and rejuvenation.

Stretching

Stretching is crucial for maintaining flexibility, improving range of motion, and preventing injuries. Post-exercise stretching can also alleviate muscle tightness and promote relaxation.

Types of Stretching:

- **Static Stretching**: Holding a stretch for 15-60 seconds can help elongate muscles and relieve tension.
- **Dynamic Stretching**: Involves controlled movements that prepare muscles for subsequent activity, which can be useful both pre- and post-exercise.
- **Proprioceptive Neuromuscular Facilitation (PNF)**: A more advanced form of stretching that involves both stretching and contracting the muscle group being targeted.

Incorporating stretching into a daily routine can significantly enhance recovery and overall athletic performance.

Yoga

Yoga combines stretching, strength, and mindfulness, offering a comprehensive approach to recovery. The practice of yoga enhances flexibility, reduces stress, and improves overall body awareness.

Benefits of Yoga for Recovery:

- **Flexibility**: Regular practice can improve the flexibility of muscles and joints, aiding in recovery.
- **Breathing Techniques**: Yoga promotes deep, mindful breathing, which can enhance oxygen delivery to muscles and reduce stress.
- **Stress Reduction**: The meditative aspect of yoga helps in managing stress, which is crucial for recovery.

Integrating yoga sessions into a weekly routine can provide significant benefits, both physically and mentally.

Massage

Massage therapy can help reduce muscle tension, improve circulation, and accelerate the removal of metabolic waste products from the muscles. Regular massage sessions can enhance recovery by addressing muscle imbalances and promoting relaxation.

Types of Massage:

- **Swedish Massage**: Uses long, flowing strokes to improve circulation and relax muscles.
- **Deep Tissue Massage**: Targets deeper layers of muscle tissue to alleviate chronic tension and improve muscle function.
- **Sports Massage**: Specifically designed for athletes, focusing on areas of the body that are overused and stressed from repetitive

movements.

Incorporating massage into a recovery regimen can help maintain muscle health and prevent injuries.

Ice Baths

My favourite! Ice baths, or cold-water immersion, involve submerging the body in cold water for a short period. This method can reduce inflammation, numb pain, and enhance recovery.

Benefits of Ice Baths:

- **Reduced Inflammation**: Cold exposure constricts blood vessels, reducing swelling and inflammation.
- **Pain Relief**: The numbing effect of cold water can alleviate soreness and discomfort.
- **Improved Recovery**: By reducing inflammation and pain, ice baths can expedite the recovery process.

To maximize benefits, ice baths should be taken shortly after intense training sessions, with a typical duration of 10-15 minutes.

Contrast Showers

Contrast showers involve alternating between hot and cold water, which can stimulate blood flow and enhance recovery.

How Contrast Showers Work:

- **Hot Water**: Dilates blood vessels, promoting circulation and

relaxation.
- **Cold Water**: Constricts blood vessels, reducing inflammation and swelling.

A typical contrast shower session might involve 3-4 cycles of hot (2-3 minutes) and cold (30 seconds to 1 minute) water. This method can invigorate the body and aid in the recovery process.

Sauna

Saunas expose the body to high temperatures, promoting relaxation, sweating, and improved circulation. The heat can help relax muscles, reduce stiffness, and enhance overall recovery.

Benefits of Saunas:

- **Muscle Relaxation**: Heat helps to relax tense muscles, reducing soreness.
- **Detoxification**: Sweating can help remove toxins from the body.
- **Improved Circulation**: Increased heart rate and blood flow can promote healing and recovery.

Regular sauna sessions, especially following intense workouts, can support muscle recovery and overall well-being.

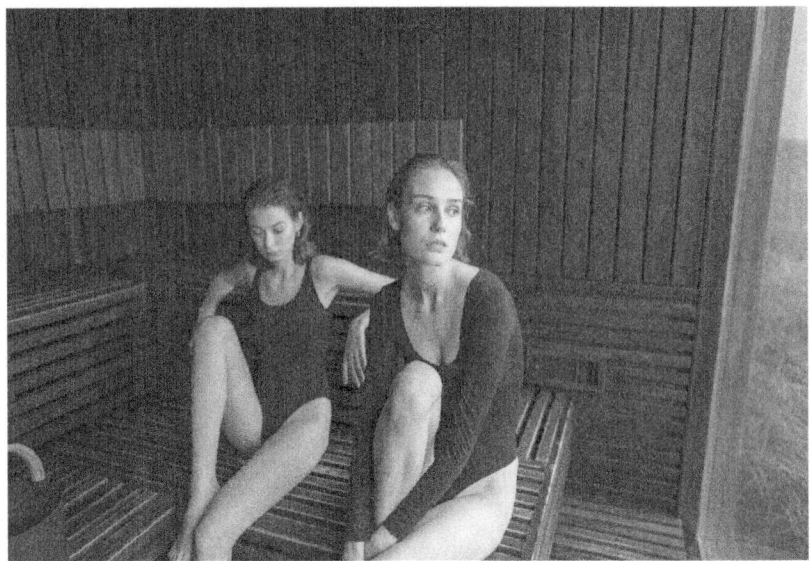

Hydration

Proper hydration is essential for optimal recovery. Water plays a crucial role in maintaining bodily functions, including temperature regulation, nutrient transport, and waste removal.

Hydration Tips:

- **Drink Regularly**: Consuming water throughout the day, not just during and after workouts, ensures consistent hydration.
- **Electrolytes**: Replenishing electrolytes lost through sweat is vital. This can be achieved through sports drinks or natural sources like coconut water.
- **Monitor Urine Colour**: Light-coloured urine typically indicates good hydration, while dark urine suggests the need for more fluids.

Maintaining adequate hydration supports muscle function, reduces the risk of cramps, and enhances overall recovery.

Delayed Onset Muscle Soreness (DOMS)

DOMS is the muscle pain and stiffness that occurs typically 24-72 hours after strenuous exercise. It results from microtraumas in muscle fibers during intense or unfamiliar physical activity.

Managing DOMS:

- **Active Recovery**: Light exercise can help alleviate DOMS by promoting blood flow to affected muscles.
- **Stretching and Yoga**: Gentle stretching and yoga can relieve muscle tightness associated with DOMS.
- **Massage**: Can help reduce muscle stiffness and enhance recovery.
- **Hydration and Nutrition**: Proper hydration and consuming anti-inflammatory foods (e.g., berries, nuts) can aid in reducing DOMS.
- **Cold Therapy**: Ice baths and cold packs can help mitigate inflammation and soreness.

Understanding and managing DOMS is crucial for maintaining consistent training schedules and avoiding prolonged discomfort.

8

Injuries

Training for a 100-mile trek is a demanding endevour that places significant stress on various parts of the body, particularly the ankles, feet, and knees. These areas are prone to specific injuries due to repetitive strain, uneven terrains, and the sheer physical toll of long-distance hiking. Understanding these injuries, their treatment, and when to seek professional help is crucial for successful training and a safe trek.

Ankle Injuries
1. Sprains
Ankle sprains are common injuries that occur when the ligaments supporting the ankle stretch beyond their limits and tear. This can happen from missteps, uneven surfaces, or sudden twists.

Symptoms: Pain, swelling, bruising, and instability of the ankle.

Treatment:

- **Rest**: Avoid putting weight on the injured ankle.

- **Ice**: Apply ice packs for 15-20 minutes every 2-3 hours during the first 48 hours.
- **Compression**: Use an elastic bandage to reduce swelling.
- **Elevation**: Keep the ankle elevated above heart level to decrease swelling.
- **Rehabilitation**: Gradually introduce exercises to restore range of motion, strength, and stability.

When to Seek Professional Help: If pain and swelling are severe, or if you cannot bear weight on the ankle, consult a healthcare provider. Persistent instability or pain after initial treatment may require professional evaluation and possibly imaging studies.

2. Achilles Tendinitis

Achilles tendinitis is an overuse injury of the Achilles tendon, which connects the calf muscles to the heel bone.

Symptoms: Pain and stiffness along the Achilles tendon, especially in the morning or after activity.

Treatment:

- **Rest**: Limit activities that exacerbate pain.
- **Ice**: Apply ice to reduce inflammation and pain.
- **Stretching**: Gentle stretching of the calf muscles can help.
- **Orthotics**: Use supportive footwear or orthotic inserts.
- **Physical Therapy**: Specific exercises to strengthen the calf muscles and improve tendon flexibility.

When to Seek Professional Help: If pain persists despite rest and conservative treatments, or if there is significant swelling or a palpable lump on the tendon, seek medical advice. Persistent or severe symptoms may indicate a partial tear, requiring professional intervention.

Foot Injuries

1. **Plantar Fasciitis**

Plantar fasciitis involves inflammation of the plantar fascia, a thick band of tissue that runs across the bottom of the foot.

Symptoms: Sharp pain in the heel or arch of the foot, typically worse in the morning or after prolonged periods of standing or walking.

Treatment:

- **Rest**: Reduce activities that trigger pain.
- **Ice**: Apply ice to the affected area for 15-20 minutes several times a day.
- **Stretching**: Stretching exercises for the Achilles tendon and plantar fascia.
- **Supportive Footwear**: Shoes with good arch support and cushioning.
- **Orthotics**: Custom orthotic devices can provide additional support.

When to Seek Professional Help: If pain is severe or persists despite home treatment, consult a healthcare provider. Persistent symptoms may benefit from more advanced treatments such as physical therapy, steroid injections, or, in rare cases, surgery.

2. **Blisters**

Blisters are fluid-filled sacs that form on the skin due to friction, often from ill-fitting footwear.

Symptoms: Painful, raised areas of skin filled with clear fluid.

Treatment:

- **Prevention**: Wear well-fitted, moisture-wicking socks and properly fitting footwear.
- **Protection**: Use blister pads or moleskin to protect vulnerable areas.
- **Care**: If a blister forms, keep it clean and covered. If necessary, drain it with a sterilized needle, but do not remove the skin.

When to Seek Professional Help: Seek medical attention if blisters show signs of infection (redness, warmth, pus) or if they are extensive and severely painful.

Knee Injuries

. 1. Patellofemoral Pain Syndrome (Runner's Knee)

This condition involves pain around the kneecap, often due to overuse, misalignment, or muscular imbalances.

Symptoms: Pain around or behind the kneecap, especially when walking, running, or descending stairs.

Treatment:

- **Rest**: Avoid activities that aggravate the pain.
- **Ice**: Apply ice packs to reduce pain and inflammation.
- **Compression**: Use knee supports or braces if necessary.

- **Exercise**: Strengthen the quadriceps, hamstrings, and hip muscles. Stretching can also help.
- **Footwear**: Ensure proper footwear to avoid excessive stress on the knee.

When to Seek Professional Help: If pain persists or worsens despite conservative measures, consult a healthcare provider. Persistent or severe symptoms may require physical therapy or further evaluation.

2. Iliotibial (IT) Band Syndrome

IT band syndrome occurs when the iliotibial band, a ligament that runs along the outside of the thigh, becomes tight or inflamed.

Symptoms: Pain on the outer side of the knee, which may worsen with activity.

Treatment:

- **Rest**: Reduce activities that cause pain.
- **Ice**: Apply ice to the affected area.
- **Stretching**: Stretch the IT band and surrounding muscles.
- **Foam Rolling**: Use a foam roller to massage and loosen the IT band.
- **Strengthening**: Strengthen hip and thigh muscles to reduce strain on the IT band.

When to Seek Professional Help: If pain persists despite self-care, consult a healthcare provider. Physical therapy may be necessary to address underlying biomechanical issues.

General Advice on When To Seek Professional Help

- **Persistent Pain**: Any pain that does not improve with rest and home treatment within a reasonable period (usually a few days to a week) should be evaluated by a professional.
- **Severe Symptoms**: Severe pain, significant swelling, inability to bear weight, or visible deformity requires immediate medical attention.
- **Recurring Injuries**: Recurrent injuries indicate that there may be an underlying issue, such as improper training technique, biomechanical abnormalities, or inadequate footwear, that needs professional assessment and correction.
- **Infection Signs**: Redness, warmth, pus, or fever in conjunction with an injury suggests infection and requires prompt medical evaluation.

9

General Advice on When to Seek Professional Help

- **Persistent Pain**: Any pain that does not improve with rest and home treatment within a reasonable period (usually a few days to a week) should be evaluated by a professional.
- **Severe Symptoms**: Severe pain, significant swelling, inability to bear weight, or visible deformity requires immediate medical attention.
- **Recurring Injuries**: Recurrent injuries indicate that there may be an underlying issue, such as improper training technique, biomechanical abnormalities, or inadequate footwear, that needs professional assessment and correction.
- **Infection Signs**: Redness, warmth, pus, or fever in conjunction with an injury suggests infection and requires prompt medical evaluation.

10

Training Programme

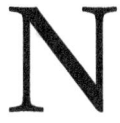ow, with this wealth of background knowledge, we are headed into the actual six week programme.

Week 1

This is the start!

These workouts are fairly easy and are a good break in.

Don't go all out on them. It's easy to be so motivated that you go at it 120%. Getting hurt now wont help you get to Fort William. So, relax into it and enjoy it. Your goal is to complete all the workout and to find your training weight on kettlebells as well as pace on step ups.

Monday
   Warm up - 3 rounds of (5 squats, 5 calf raises, 5 toe touches, 5 lunge stretches);
   Step ups - 600 step ups with a 30lb pack;
   Calf raises (unloaded) - (20 seconds activity, 10 seconds hold in up

position) x 8 rounds

Cool down - foam roll legs and lower back

Tuesday

Warm up - walk 800m or half a mile. Work on hip rotations, slow squats, lunges and windmills for the upper body.

Kettlebells or dumbbells - 3 rounds of goblet squats, swings, overhead press, bend row, step back lunges and calf raises. 8 to 12 reps on each.

Walk or run for 20 minutes. If you have access to and prefer, then you could row or bike. Keep the pace moderate.

Plank - 3 x 60s planks. Go onto your knees when you have to but complete each 60s plank before resting.

Try following an online yoga video to cool down. No more than 20 min duration.

Wednesday

Ruck 2 miles with a 30lb pack. Easy pace. Get used to moving.

Thursday

Warm up - 3 rounds of (5 squats, 5 calf raises, 5 toe touches, 5 lunge stretches);

Step ups - 650 step ups with a 30lb pack;

Calf raises (unloaded) - (20 seconds activity, 10 seconds hold in up position) x 8 rounds

Cool down - foam roll legs and lower back

Friday

Warm up - walk 800m or half a mile. Work on hip rotations, slow squats, lunges and windmills for the upper body.

Kettlebells or dumbbells - 3 rounds of goblet squats, swings, overhead press, bend row, step back lunges and calf raises. 8 to 12 reps on each.

Walk or run for 20 minutes. If you have access to and prefer, then you could row or bike. Keep the pace moderate.

Plank - 3 x 60s planks. Go onto your knees when you have to but complete each 60s plank before resting.

Try following an online yoga video to cool down. No more than 20 min duration.

Saturday

Ruck 7 miles with the pack and kit you will do The West Highland Way in. Throw in some tins of food to account for a few days' food. Keep the pace slow and measured. Stay hydrated. Watch for blisters.

Sunday

REST. no activity. Go for a light walk or other active recovery. If you stretch then fine. If you do yoga, ensure it's not ashtanga or hot yoga. Rest. Recover.

Week 2

This is a good week. You may be feeling a bit sore from last week but you did all you could to recover on Sunday didn't you?

You may experience DOMS or have experienced it last week. Follow the guidance in this guide and it will help tremendously.

This week you start to use sandbags to train with. These are great for building your overall strength and your core as well.

Monday

Warm up - 3 rounds of (5 squats, 5 calf raises, 5 toe touches, 5 lunge stretches);

Step ups - 700 step ups with a 30lb pack;

Calf raises (unloaded) - (20 seconds activity, 10 seconds hold in up position) x 8 rounds

Cool down - foam roll legs and lower back

Tuesday

Warm up - walk 800m or half a mile. Work on hip rotations, slow squats, lunges and windmills for the upper body.

Sandbag - 3 rounds of cleans, overhead press, bent row, high pulls, front squat, lunges and overhead squat. 8 to 12 reps on each.

Walk or run for 20 minutes. If you have access to and prefer, then you could row or bike. Keep the pace moderate.

Plank - 3 x 60s planks. Go onto your knees when you have to but complete each 60s plank before resting.

Try following an online yoga video to cool down. No more than 20 min duration.

Wednesday

Ruck 3 miles with a 30lb pack. Easy pace. Get used to moving.

Thursday

Warm up - 3 rounds of (5 squats, 5 calf raises, 5 toe touches, 5 lunge stretches);

Step ups - 750 step ups with a 30lb pack;

Calf raises (unloaded) - (20 seconds activity, 10 seconds hold in up position) x 8 rounds

Cool down - foam roll legs and lower back

Friday

Warm up - walk 800m or half a mile. Work on hip rotations, slow squats, lunges and windmills for the upper body.

Sandbag - 3 rounds of cleans, overhead press, bent row, high pulls, front squat, lunges and overhead squat. 8 to 12 reps on each.

Walk or run for 20 minutes. If you have access to and prefer, then you could row or bike. Keep the pace moderate.

Plank - 3 x 60s planks. Go onto your knees when you have to but complete each 60s plank before resting.

Try following an online yoga video to cool down. No more than 20 min duration.

Saturday

Ruck 8 miles with the pack and kit you will do The West Highland Way in. Throw in some tins of food to account for a few days' food. Keep the pace slow and measured. Stay hydrated. Watch for blisters.

Sunday

REST. no activity. Go for a light walk or other active recovery. If you stretch then fine. If you do yoga, ensure it's not ashtanga or hot yoga. Rest. Recover.

Week 3

You are half way there now. You will notice a difference in energy levels. You are stronger. Possibly leaner.

Keep going!

Monday

Warm up - 3 rounds of (5 squats, 5 calf raises, 5 toe touches, 5 lunge stretches);

Step ups - 800 step ups with a 35lb pack;

Calf raises (unloaded) - (20 seconds activity, 10 seconds hold in up position) x 8 rounds

Cool down - foam roll legs and lower back

Tuesday

Warm up - walk 800m or half a mile. Work on hip rotations, slow squats, lunges and windmills for the upper body.

Kettlebells or dumbbells - 3 rounds of goblet squats, swings, overhead press, bend row, step back lunges and calf raises. 12 to 15 reps on each.

Walk or run for 20 minutes. If you have access to and prefer, then you could row or bike. Keep the pace moderate.

Plank - 3 x 60s planks. Go onto your knees when you have to but complete each 60s plank before resting.

Try following an online yoga video to cool down. No more than 20 min duration.

Wednesday

Ruck 4 miles with a 40lb pack. Easy pace. Get used to moving.

Thursday

Warm up - 3 rounds of (5 squats, 5 calf raises, 5 toe touches, 5 lunge stretches);

Step ups - 850 step ups with a 35lb pack;

Calf raises (unloaded) - (20 seconds activity, 10 seconds hold in up position) x 8 rounds

Cool down - foam roll legs and lower back

Friday

Warm up - walk 800m or half a mile. Work on hip rotations, slow squats, lunges and windmills for the upper body.

Kettlebells or dumbbells - 3 rounds of goblet squats, swings, overhead press, bend row, step back lunges and calf raises. 12 to 15 reps on each.

Walk or run for 20 minutes. If you have access to and prefer, then you could row or bike. Keep the pace moderate.

Plank - 3 x 60s planks. Go onto your knees when you have to but complete each 60s plank before resting.

Try following an online yoga video to cool down. No more than 20 min duration.

Saturday

Ruck 9 miles with the pack and kit you will do The West Highland Way in. Throw in some tins of food to account for a few days' food. Keep the pace slow and measured. Stay hydrated. Watch for blisters.

Sunday

REST. no activity. Go for a light walk or other active recovery. If you stretch then fine. If you do yoga, ensure it's not ashtanga or hot yoga. Rest. Recover.

Week 4

You've been grinding now for a month. Its impressive. Your pack will feel better. You'll be good at walking in various kinds of weather. Your legs are now a lot stronger and mentally you are more resilient. There's a bigger increase in distance on Saturdays ruck as well.

Monday

Warm up - 3 rounds of (5 squats, 5 calf raises, 5 toe touches, 5 lunge stretches);

Step ups - 900 step ups with a 30lb pack;

Calf raises (unloaded) - (20 seconds activity, 10 seconds hold in up position) x 8 rounds

Cool down - foam roll legs and lower back

Tuesday

Warm up - walk 800m or half a mile. Work on hip rotations, slow squats, lunges and windmills for the upper body.

Sandbag - 3 rounds of cleans, overhead press, bent row, high pulls, front squat, lunges and overhead squat. 12 to 15 reps on each.

Walk or run for 20 minutes. If you have access to and prefer, then you could row or bike. Keep the pace moderate.

Plank - 3 x 60s planks. Go onto your knees when you have to but complete each 60s plank before resting.

Try following an online yoga video to cool down. No more than 20 min duration.

Wednesday

Ruck 5 miles with a 40lb pack. Easy pace. Get used to moving.

Thursday

Warm up - 3 rounds of (5 squats, 5 calf raises, 5 toe touches, 5 lunge stretches);

Step ups - 950 step ups with a 30lb pack;

Calf raises (unloaded) - (20 seconds activity, 10 seconds hold in up position) x 8 rounds

Cool down - foam roll legs and lower back

Friday

Warm up - walk 800m or half a mile. Work on hip rotations, slow squats, lunges and windmills for the upper body.

Sandbag - 3 rounds of cleans, overhead press, bent row, high pulls, front squat, lunges and overhead squat. 12 to 15 reps on each.

Walk or run for 20 minutes. If you have access to and prefer, then you could row or bike. Keep the pace moderate.

Plank - 3 x 60s planks. Go onto your knees when you have to but complete each 60s plank before resting.

Try following an online yoga video to cool down. No more than 20 min duration.

Saturday

Ruck 11 miles with the pack and kit you will do The West Highland Way in. Throw in some tins of food to account for a few days' food. Keep the pace slow and measured. Stay hydrated. Watch for blisters.

Sunday

REST. no activity. Go for a light walk or other active recovery. If you stretch then fine. If you do yoga, ensure it's not ashtanga or hot yoga. Rest. Recover.

Week 5

This is the highest volume week. Stay strong. Keep deliberate. Focus on your recovery, hydration and nutrition.

Monday

Warm up - 3 rounds of (5 squats, 5 calf raises, 5 toe touches, 5 lunge stretches);

Step ups - 1,000 step ups with a 30lb pack;

Calf raises (unloaded) - (20 seconds activity, 10 seconds hold in up position) x 8 rounds

Cool down - foam roll legs and lower back

Tuesday

Warm up - walk 800m or half a mile. Work on hip rotations, slow squats, lunges and windmills for the upper body.

Kettlebells or dumbbells - 3 rounds of goblet squats, swings, overhead press, bend row, step back lunges and calf raises. 12 to 15 reps on each.

Walk or run for 20 minutes. If you have access to and prefer, then you could row or bike. Keep the pace moderate.

Plank - 3 x 60s planks. Go onto your knees when you have to but complete each 60s plank before resting.

Try following an online yoga video to cool down. No more than 20 min duration.

Wednesday

Ruck 6 miles with a 40lb pack. Easy pace. Get used to moving.

Thursday

Warm up - 3 rounds of (5 squats, 5 calf raises, 5 toe touches, 5 lunge stretches);

Step ups - 1,100 step ups with a 30lb pack;

Calf raises (unloaded) - (20 seconds activity, 10 seconds hold in up position) x 8 rounds

Cool down - foam roll legs and lower back

Friday

Warm up - walk 800m or half a mile. Work on hip rotations, slow squats, lunges and windmills for the upper body.

Kettlebells or dumbbells - 3 rounds of goblet squats, swings, overhead press, bend row, step back lunges and calf raises. 12 to 15 reps on each.

Walk or run for 20 minutes. If you have access to and prefer, then you could row or bike. Keep the pace moderate.

Plank - 3 x 60s planks. Go onto your knees when you have to but complete each 60s plank before resting.

Try following an online yoga video to cool down. No more than 20 min duration.

Saturday

Ruck 12 miles with the pack and kit you will do The West Highland Way in. Throw in some tins of food to account for a few days' food. Keep the pace slow and measured. Stay hydrated. Watch for blisters.

Sunday

REST. no activity. Go for a light walk or other active recovery. If you stretch then fine. If you do yoga, ensure it's not ashtanga or hot yoga. Rest. Recover.

Week 6

The final week. The loads ease slightly so you are fully recovered going into The West Highland Way.

Monday

Warm up - 3 rounds of (5 squats, 5 calf raises, 5 toe touches, 5 lunge stretches);

Step ups - 1,000 step ups with a 30lb pack;

Calf raises (unloaded) - (20 seconds activity, 10 seconds hold in up position) x 8 rounds

Cool down - foam roll legs and lower back

Tuesday

Warm up - walk 800m or half a mile. Work on hip rotations, slow squats, lunges and windmills for the upper body.

Sandbag - 3 rounds of cleans, overhead press, bent row, high pulls, front squat, lunges and overhead squat. 12 to 15 reps on each.

Walk or run for 20 minutes. If you have access to and prefer, then you could row or bike. Keep the pace moderate.

Plank - 3 x 60s planks. Go onto your knees when you have to but complete each 60s plank before resting.

Try following an online yoga video to cool down. No more than 20 min duration.

Wednesday

Ruck 6 miles with a 35lb pack. Easy pace. Get used to moving.

Thursday

Warm up - 3 rounds of (5 squats, 5 calf raises, 5 toe touches, 5 lunge stretches);

Step ups - 1,100 step ups with a 30lb pack;

Calf raises (unloaded) - (20 seconds activity, 10 seconds hold in up position) x 8 rounds

Cool down - foam roll legs and lower back

Friday

Warm up - walk 800m or half a mile. Work on hip rotations, slow squats, lunges and windmills for the upper body.

Sandbag - 3 rounds of cleans, overhead press, bent row, high pulls, front squat, lunges and overhead squat. 12 to 15 reps on each.

Walk or run for 20 minutes. If you have access to and prefer, then you could row or bike. Keep the pace moderate.

Plank - 3 x 60s planks. Go onto your knees when you have to but complete each 60s plank before resting.

Try following an online yoga video to cool down. No more than 20 min duration.

Saturday

Ruck 11 miles with the pack and kit you will do The West Highland

Way in. Throw in some tins of food to account for a few days' food. Keep the pace slow and measured. Stay hydrated. Watch for blisters.

Sunday

REST. no activity. Go for a light walk or other active recovery. If you stretch then fine. If you do yoga, ensure it's not ashtanga or hot yoga. Rest. Recover.

11

Conclusion

There you have it! All the info you need for getting fit for The West Highland Way or similar.

If you have enjoyed this book and you got something from it, I would really appreciate you heading over to Amazon and leaving a review. Thanks and happy hiking!

CONCLUSION

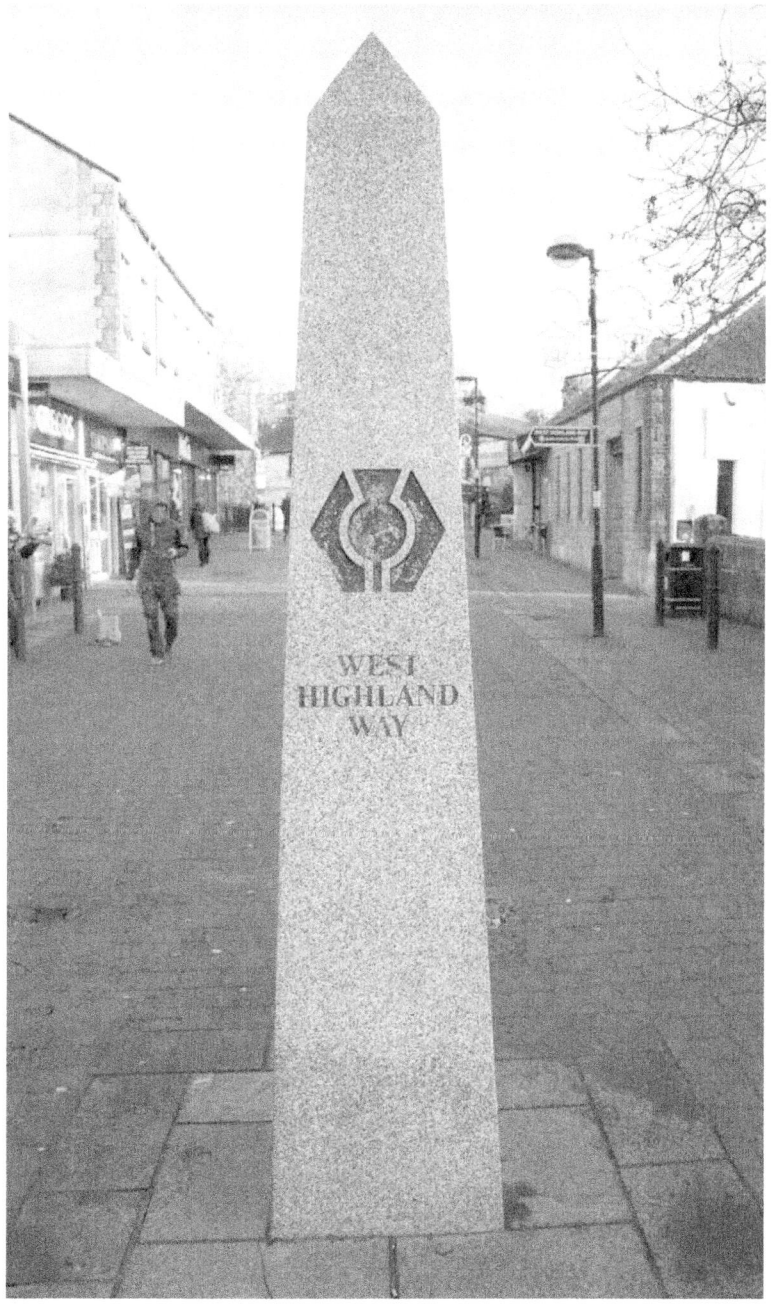

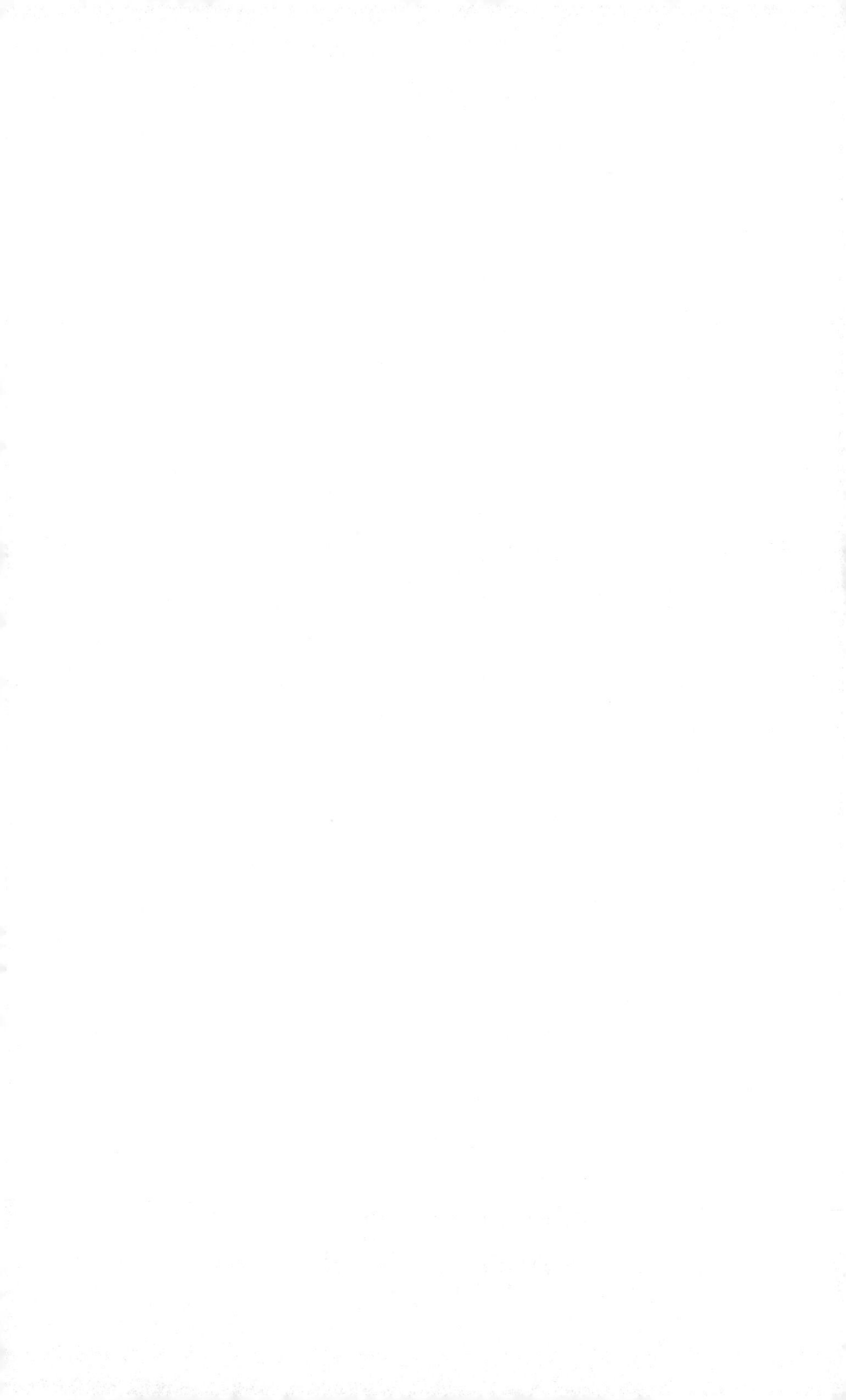

Printed in Great Britain
by Amazon